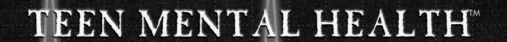

TEEN MENTAL HEALTH™

conduct
disorder

Barbara Gottfried Hollander

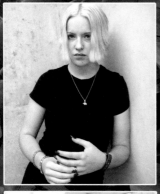

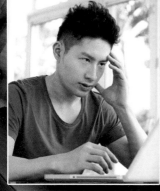

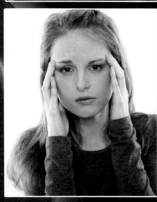

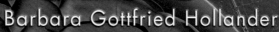

ROSEN
PUBLISHING®

New York

Published in 2014 by The Rosen Publishing Group, Inc.
29 East 21st Street, New York, NY 10010

Library of Congress Cataloging-in-Publication Data

Hollander, Barbara Gottfried.
Conduct disorder/Barbara Gottfried Hollander.
    pages cm.—(Teen mental health)
Includes bibliographical references and index.
ISBN 978-1-4777-1752-3 (library binding)
1. Conduct disorders in adolescence. 2. Juvenile delinquency. I. Title.
RJ506.C65H65 2014
618.9285'81—dc23

2013021770

Manufactured in the United States of America

CPSIA Compliance Information: Batch #W14YA: For further information, contact Rosen Publishing, New York, New York, at 1-800-237-9932.

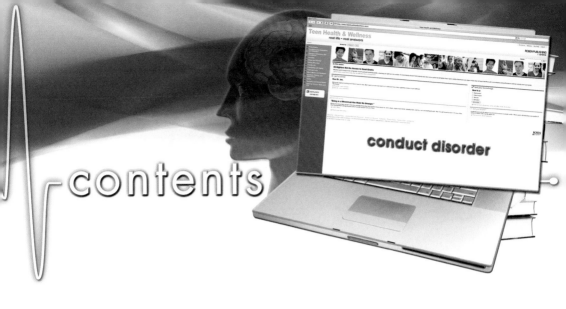

contents

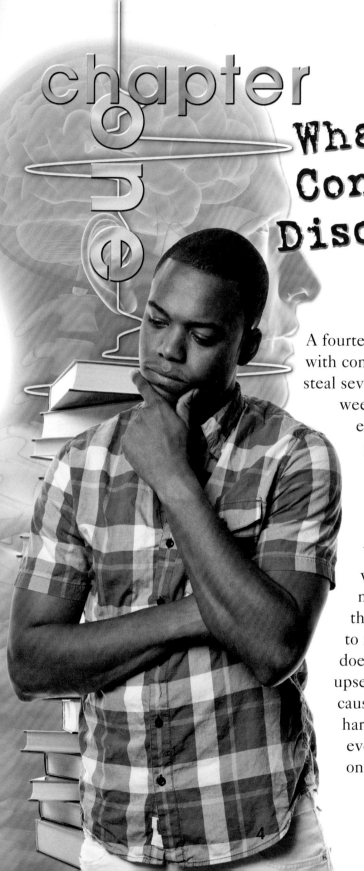

chapter one

What Is Conduct Disorder?

A fourteen-year-old boy with conduct disorder may steal several times in one week. He can repeatedly lie to his parents about his actions, skip school, and torture the neighbor's dog. When confronted with the seriousness of his actions, the teen shows little to no remorse. He does not appear sad, upset, or apologetic for causing physical harm. This teen may even set his house on fire. Again, no remorse is shown for these actions.

Threatening people, harming animals, and destroying property over and over again are often signs of a mental condition called conduct disorder (CD). According to the *Encyclopedia of Mental Disorders*, this mental condition affects 9 percent of male and 2 percent of female children and teens. It is frequently visible by the age of ten. Children with conduct disorder violate the basic rights of others. They carry out their destructive and disruptive behaviors at school, home, or in other settings. This troublesome behavior makes it difficult for them to form and maintain relationships with friends and family.

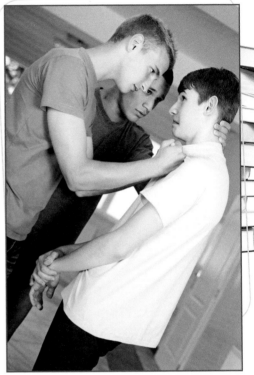

Teens who have conduct disorder usually exhibit aggressive behavior, such as intimidating and bullying others.

When a teen has an ear infection, the doctor prescribes antibiotics. The medicine treats the bacterial infection and helps the patient heal. But what about a mental illness like CD? Is there a medicine that will heal this condition? No. Mental illnesses, or serious emotional and behavioral problems, are very difficult to treat. Doctors, such as psychiatrists and neurologists, examine possible causes to determine the most appropriate treatment plans. So what causes teens to behave in destructive and cruel ways?

Is the Body Responsible?

There are several physical factors that could cause or increase the likelihood of conduct disorder. Like some other mental, emotional, and behavioral disorders, CD is more common in boys than girls. This aspect would suggest a possible genetic (or inherited) cause.

Disorders more prevalent in boys than girls include:

- Conduct disorder (CD)
- Oppositional deviant disorder (ODD)
- Attention-deficit/hyperactivity disorder (ADHD)
- Pervasive developmental disorder (autism)
- Tourette's syndrome (which includes vocal or other physical tics)

Doctors have also examined neurological, or brain-related, causes and effects. The frontal lobe of your brain (also called the cerebral cortex) is located at the top of your head and behind your forehead. It is responsible for decision making and emotions, such as empathy (or being able to relate to someone else's feelings). This part of the brain also allows you to learn from negative consequences and stay out of harm's way, like not directly touching a hot pan twice. The connection between the frontal lobe and conduct disorder also suggests that children born with brain damage to the frontal lobe may be more likely to

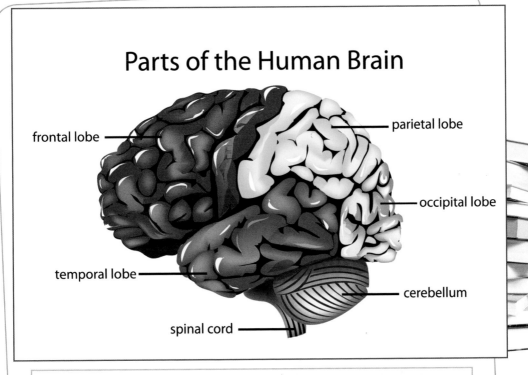

Parts of the Human Brain

frontal lobe

parietal lobe

occipital lobe

temporal lobe

cerebellum

spinal cord

A link between conduct disorder and the impairment of the brain's frontal lobe may exist.

exhibit symptoms of this disorder. Damage to the frontal lobe impairs (harms or weakens) the neurological tools needed to behave appropriately.

How might this impairment present itself in the behavior of teens? Conduct disorder affects a teen's ability to feel regret for his or her actions, like torturing an animal or setting a fire. A teen who has conduct disorder has difficulty relating to the feelings of an abused animal or a person with hurt feelings. Even the yelps of the dog or a person's tears might not cause a person with CD to feel empathy. This lack of empathy can also cause these teens to repeatedly hurt others and destroy property because they do not fully understand the repercussions of their actions or feel bad about them. Conduct disorder is marked by repeated and consistent destructive behavior.

Do Surroundings Count?

Children often model their parents' behaviors. Suppose that a teen's father is both verbally abusive (making insults and threats) and physically abusive (hitting). In this setting, the teen is more likely to become a verbal and physical abuser himself. Children who grow up with domestic violence frequently imitate the behavior of their abusive parents. Just as a parent hurts the teen, the teen hurts others. Aggressive and abusive parenting, especially by fathers, can increase the likelihood of developing CD.

If a child grows up with a parent who suffers from a mental disorder, such as antisocial personality disorder, he or she is also more likely to exhibit conduct disorder. Antisocial personality disorder involves a history of manipulating, taking advantage of, and violating others' rights. For example, suppose that a teen witnesses his father consistently manipulating his mother. The dad uses the mom to get things for himself, such as material goods or more control of the family.

Now suppose that this dad makes the following conditional statement to his wife: "I will not get angry if you stop seeing your friends." The mom is being asked to give up her friendships in return for her husband no longer getting angry. The dad is also trying to gain greater control over his family by isolating his wife. Two things can happen next: (1) The mom does not give up her friends and the next time that dad explodes, he blames her; or (2) she gives up her friends. The next time dad explodes, he finds another reason to blame mom (or one of the children). Either way, the dad explodes and blames someone else for his behavior.

Now consider the effect on the teen who has CD. He views his dad's manipulative behavior as effective. Dad

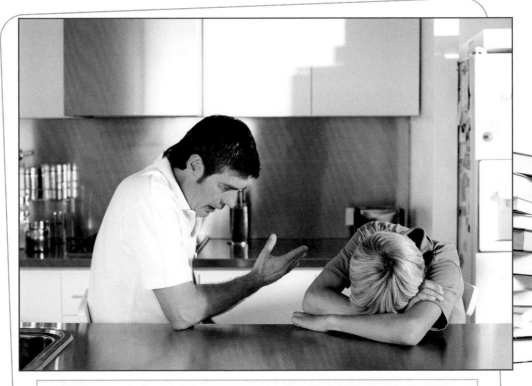

Children who come from abusive homes are more likely to have mental, emotional, and behavioral disorders.

often gets what he wants within the home environment. So the teen uses manipulation to get what he wants, too. The teen also rationalizes his physical aggression by blaming others. For example, the teen hits his mother and blames her for these actions. By imitating his father's behavior, the teen exhibits symptoms of conduct disorder consistent with violating the rights of others.

What if there are no negative repercussions for the teen's abusive behavior? What if he is given "rewards," such as getting what he wants or positive reinforcement from his father? Then the teen with CD is more likely to continue. Parents who engage in criminal behavior also put their children at a higher risk for CD by modeling destructive behavior. Alcohol and other drug addictions increase this risk, too, because they create unstable home environments and involve dysfunctional behavioral patterns.

Finally, poverty and location are other environmental factors that increase the likelihood of conduct disorder. Children who don't have enough money to afford basic needs, such as food and clothing, are more likely to present destructive behaviors that harm others. According to the article "Poverty, Social Inequality and Mental Health" by Vijaya Murali and Femi Oyebode, "Children in the poorest households are three times more likely to have a mental illness than children in the best-off households... In the behavioral domain, conduct disorder and attention-deficit/hyperactivity disorder show links with family poverty." Research also shows that children in cities, rather than rural areas, are more likely to have CD.

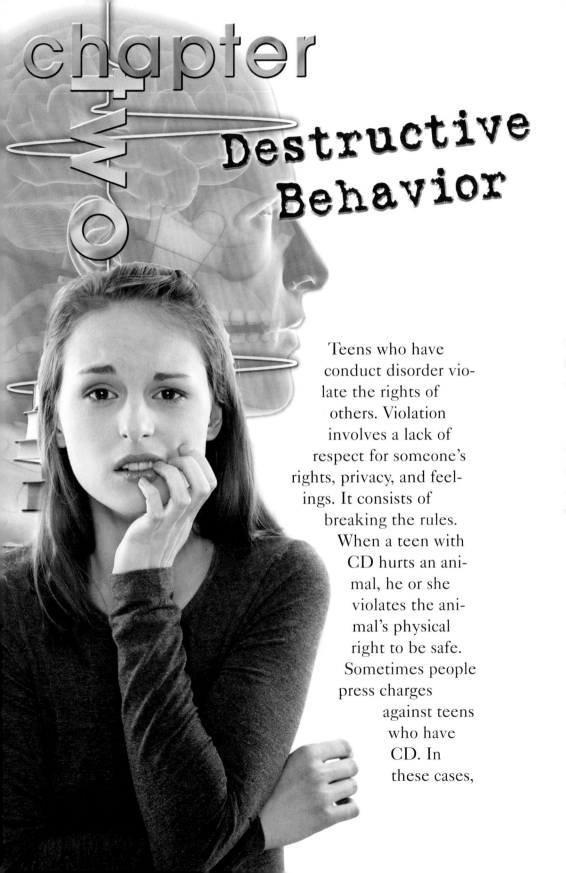

chapter two

Destructive Behavior

Teens who have conduct disorder violate the rights of others. Violation involves a lack of respect for someone's rights, privacy, and feelings. It consists of breaking the rules. When a teen with CD hurts an animal, he or she violates the animal's physical right to be safe. Sometimes people press charges against teens who have CD. In these cases, teens with conduct disorder can face jail time for criminal acts, such as murder or rape.

Hurting others can begin as thoughts. Allen Frances and Ruth Ross wrote a book about conduct disorder case studies. The book discusses a boy, Robert, who thought that "killing someone [meant] the police will get me and take care of me." Robert's judgment is impaired. He viewed killing someone as an option and thought the police would care for him if he chose this option. He did not consider how killing someone would affect the victim, his or her family and friends, or society. He did not even fully understand the consequences for himself.

Robert also showed other possible signs of CD. He tried to commit suicide. When his mother tried to stop him, he said, "Please let me go and jump. It will be better if I'm dead. I won't have to think. I won't have to worry. There's a better place." He blamed his mother for his latest suicide attempt, citing an argument. Robert had a history of getting into violent arguments. He stole from children at school, stayed out later than allowed, and sometimes skipped school. When he was angry, he ran away from home. He also started fires. Robert consistently violated the rights of others and broke the rules.

Conduct Disorder in the Classroom

Children and teens with CD usually exhibit many symptoms. In the classroom, they display unacceptable behaviors, such as hitting and stealing. They also continue these actions even after peers with similar behaviors have found more appropriate coping mechanisms.

For example, suppose that two students tend to storm out of the classroom when they are upset. The school psychologist talks to both boys separately. One student eventually understands that he cannot leave the classroom without permission. He finds more acceptable ways to cope with his frustration and anger, including visiting the school psychologist.

But the other student cannot stop storming out of the classroom and disrupting the class. His anger and frustration grow as the school year progresses. Eventually, this teen's outbursts include destroying school property and getting into frequent physical confrontations with his classmates. This teen is showing signs of conduct disorder. In school, children and teens with CD may seem uninterested, careless, or not concerned about their classwork. They have a higher risk for getting poor grades, repeating grade levels (such as doing tenth grade twice), and dropping out of school. These students challenge class rules and often miss assignments.

Students with CD have poor social skills. According to the National Association of School Psychologists, there are four different kinds of social skills:

- Survival skills: Listening, following directions, and talking respectfully
- Interpersonal skills: Asking permission, turn taking, and sharing
- Problem-solving skills: Expressing remorse, understanding consequences, taking ownership for actions, and making appropriate decisions

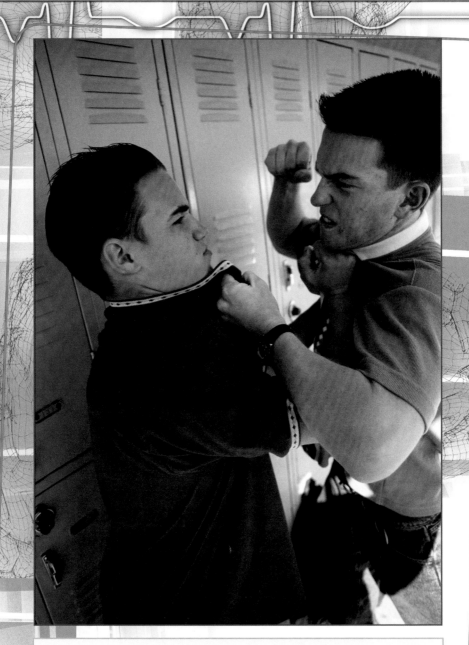

Teens with conduct disorder often get into confrontations with peers, friends, and family members.

- Conflict resolution skills: Coping with socially challenging situations, such as teasing, peer pressure, and being left out

Those with conduct disorder have trouble making friends and are often left out of social activities. This consequence can lead to other challenges, such as depression and peer groups that encourage deviant, or abnormal, behavior.

Ranges and Phases of Conduct Disorder

Children and teens exhibit different ranges of conduct disorder. Dr. Aubrey Fine notes five categories: mild (causing minor harm to other individuals), moderate, severe (causing significant harm to others), undersocialized (behavior involving violence), and socialized (behavior that includes violence in both public and private settings). She also mentions that conduct disorder may look different in boys than girls. Boys are more likely to engage in physical acts, such as fighting, stealing, and destroying property. Girls might lie, begin abusing drugs, or even engage in prostitution (the act of selling sex for money).

Children often show signs of conduct disorder in phases, with early warning signs. For example, Robert had trouble with transitions as a young child. He reacted with anger to change or discipline. He was physically aggressive, often fighting with older children. Many times, Robert was also anxious and sad. He lacked the coping skills needed for normal stressors in the house (for

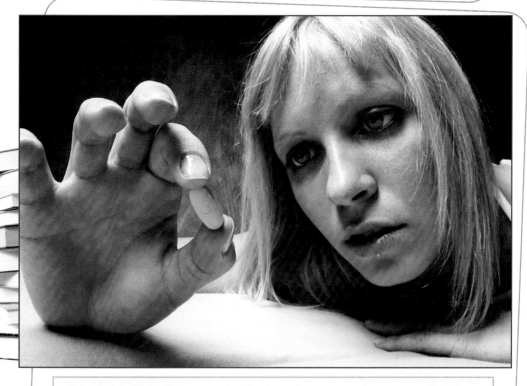

Conduct disorder may include substance abuse, such as drug and alcohol abuse.

instance, someone not giving him attention) and reacted even more negatively to bigger home challenges, such as divorce. There are many children and teens who exhibit these behaviors (being worried, sad, and even physical). Not all of these children have CD. Mental disorders are difficult to diagnose, especially in children and teens. According to Dr. Fine, between 1.3 and 3.8 million children suffer from conduct disorder.

Conduct disorder appears in stages. A young child with CD does not begin life by maliciously setting fires or robbing a store. As a child with CD grows, more deviant behaviors appear. Treatment can affect how conduct disorder progresses. A child with CD may have a greater chance at a normal life if he or she receives treatment. For example, suppose a ten-year-old boy with conduct disorder steals from other students in school. By the age of eleven, he is stealing money from his parents' wallets at home. How might treatment affect this boy's future?

Imagine that the parents and teacher work together with a psychologist to carry out consequences for the boy's behavior and help him understand why he steals. These treatment tools enable the boy to accept responsibility for his stealing, understand that his actions have consequences, and make better and healthier behavioral choices. Next, consider a boy that does not confront or deal with his stealing. He blames the teacher for his stealing, saying that she is "out to get him." He justifies stealing at home, claiming his parents don't give him the same amount of spending money that his friends get. He does not receive consequences that he equates with his actions. By the age of sixteen, this teen is shoplifting. As you will learn, treatment does not always work. But it can provide valuable tools both for the teen who has conduct disorder and his or her caregivers.

As CD develops, teens may engage in criminal activities that include the following:

- Using weapons (such as guns and knives) to seriously hurt or kill people and animals
- Robbing businesses and homes
- Mugging people (robbing someone in public)

- Extortion (use of threats to get something, i.e., blackmail)
- Forgery (falsely making a document, for instance, a fake check)
- Rape (forced sexual attack)
- Breaking into cars and homes
- Prostitution

Teens with conduct disorder can have suicidal tendencies, including fantasizing about and attempting to kill themselves. These threats should be taken seriously, with appropriate medical involvement. Teens with CD are also at a greater risk for abusing drugs, such as alcohol. According to an article in the *Archives of Pediatric and Adolescent Medicine*, there is a connection between conduct disorder in teens and substance abuse in adults. In fact, "CD is a major predictor of SUDs [substance abuse disorders] in adulthood," wrote the article's author, Dr. David W. Brook of the New York University School of Medicine in New York City.

MYTHS AND FACTS

Myth: All teens that get into physical fights have conduct disorder.

Fact: Physical fighting is a symptom of conduct disorder. However, not all teens who get into fights have conduct disorder.

Myth: Boys and girls tend to show conduct disorder in the same ways.

Fact: Boys with conduct disorder are more likely to fight, steal, and vandalize property (purposely damage and/or destroy it). Girls are more likely to lie, run away, and exchange sex for things (such as money).

Myth: Home life does not affect conduct disorder.

Fact: A challenging home life, such as an abusive environment, can increase the likelihood of developing conduct disorder.

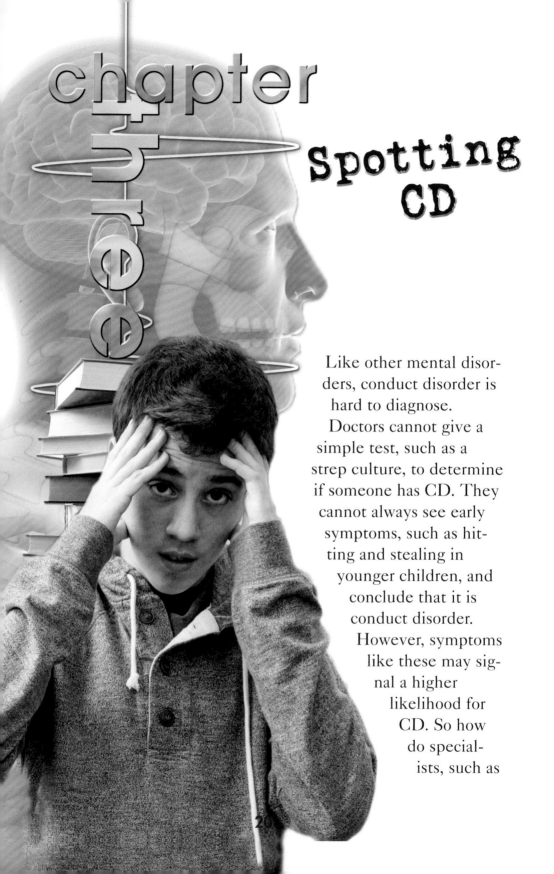

chapter three

Spotting CD

Like other mental disorders, conduct disorder is hard to diagnose. Doctors cannot give a simple test, such as a strep culture, to determine if someone has CD. They cannot always see early symptoms, such as hitting and stealing in younger children, and conclude that it is conduct disorder. However, symptoms like these may signal a higher likelihood for CD. So how do specialists, such as psychologists (people trained in dealing with the mind and emotions) and psychiatrists (people specializing in mental illnesses), diagnose conduct disorder?

Specialists rely on reports from parents, teachers, and others that describe a child or teen's behavior in different settings. Suppose that you are a teen under observation for CD. Medical professionals will ask your caregivers, teachers, and other doctors questions about you, such as:

- Do you lie?
- Do you steal?
- Do you often get into physical fights?
- Have you seriously hurt someone with a weapon?
- Do your teachers report that you are a bully?
- Are you physically cruel to animals?
- Have you ever sexually assaulted someone?
- Do you purposely destroy property?
- Do you set fires?
- Do you run away from home or skip school?
- Have you ever been arrested?
- Have you been expelled or suspended from school?
- Do you abuse drugs?
- Do you feel remorse when your actions hurt others?
- Can you relate to other people's feelings?

According to the American Psychiatric Association, conduct disorder means there is a consistent violation of others' rights or age-appropriate behavior in three or more of the following areas in the past twelve months:

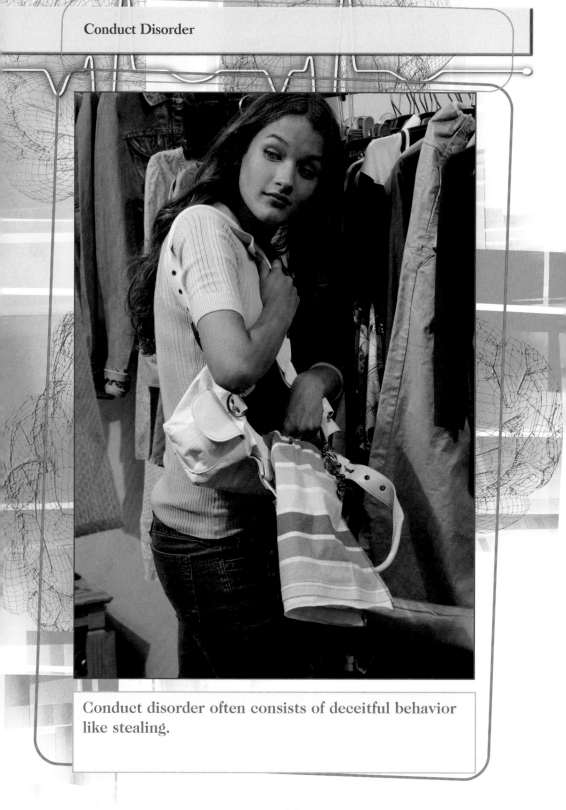

Conduct disorder often consists of deceitful behavior like stealing.

(1) aggression toward people or animals; (2) destruction of property; (3) lying or theft; and (4) serious violation of rules, such as running away from home, skipping school, or using drugs. A child or teen with CD should also have shown one of these behaviors within the past six months.

Conduct disorder involves a persistent pattern of aggression, destruction, and other violations. For example, a teen with CD *repeatedly* skips school, hurts animals, and sets fires. Many teens may engage in antisocial behavior once or a few times. For instance, suppose a high school student skips school because she wants to hang out with her college friends. Or another teen tries alcohol at a party because his friends pressure him to take a drink. These examples of risk taking do not necessarily mean the person has conduct disorder. These behaviors occurred once, not repeatedly.

To diagnose CD, medical specialists put together a psychological history of the patient. They also compare the patient's behavior to age-appropriate norms. For example, a psychiatrist records the number of patient's truancies, or unexcused absences from school. He or she may then compare it to the number of truancies for an average teen. Medical specialists consider truancy a conduct disorder symptom, particularly when children begin skipping school before the age of thirteen. But again, truancy is one possible symptom of this mental illness. There are other reasons for truancy, including the fear of being bullied or working long hours in a job while in school.

Psychiatrists put together a complete picture before making a CD diagnosis. They might also consider another mental disorder called oppositional defiant disorder (ODD). ODD is a milder form of conduct disorder and can become CD. Oppositional defiant disorder is disruptive in family, school, and social environments. Like CD, ODD also involves persistent behavior, such as repeatedly arguing with teachers or not accepting responsibility for disruptive actions. But ODD does not involve serious violations of others' rights.

Think About It

Consider when teens typically begin risky behaviors. According to the *Journal of Family Practice*, "Forty percent of adult alcoholics report having had their first alcoholism-related symptoms between ages 15 and 19." This publication also reports that gambling problems usually begin at age twelve, and three million teens contract sexually transmitted diseases. Children and teens face a lot of pressure to engage in risky behaviors. This pressure comes from home, friends, ads, and other places.

Reacting appropriately to these pressures requires a three-step thinking process: taking in the situation, processing it and deciding on a response, and carrying out an appropriate action. Impulsivity is acting without thinking. It does not include this three-step process. Impulsivity often goes with risk taking, as teens react to desires, rather than contemplate options or consequences. For example, suppose a teen's friend pressures him or her to try drugs. A three-step decision-making process might involve the following:

1) The teen hears the friend's offer to try drugs.
2) The teen weighs the pros and cons of accepting his or her friend's offer and decides it is harmful to take the drugs.
3) The teen refuses the drugs and walks away.

Children and teens with conduct disorder have a breakdown in the decision-making process. They repeatedly and impulsively react to situations without considering the consequences. Teens with normal risk behaviors exhibit moderate violations (such as skipping school once) and learn from the conse-

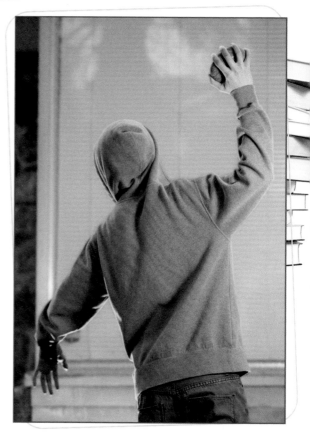

Teens with conduct disorder might impulsively destroy property.

quences (getting detention, for example). But teens with a mental illness, such as conduct disorder, show serious pathological behavior (like repeatedly skipping school), which carries more severe consequences (repeating grades, for example).

Environmental and Biological Factors

Medical specialists also examine the patient's environment when diagnosing CD. This information helps with the patient's profile and treatment plans. For example, what is the home situation? Remember that teens from abusive homes and/or poorer areas are more likely to have conduct disorder. If a psychiatrist knows that a child comes from an abusive home, he or she may better understand the teen's thought process and actions. In addition, part of the treatment plan may involve separating the child from the abusive parent. Specialists will also look at other stressors, such as divorced parents or deaths in the immediate family.

Conduct disorder involves impaired judgment. Remember that decision making is associated with the brain. A 2011 study in the United Kingdom by the Wellcome Trust and the Medical Research Council shows that regions of the brain called the amygdala and insula are smaller in teens with antisocial behavior, such as CD. These parts of the brain are associated with processing emotion and feeling empathy. A smaller insula often shows more severe behavioral problems. Sometimes brain imaging tests, such as magnetic resonance imaging (MRI) scans, may be useful in explaining symptoms of a mental disorder, particularly when a child or teen has suffered brain damage. Still, many teens with CD have normal brain imaging tests.

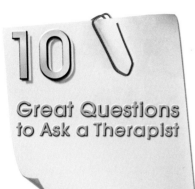

10

Great Questions to Ask a Therapist

1. Do I have conduct disorder?

2. How do I know if I have another mental disorder, like oppositional defiant disorder, that looks like conduct disorder?

3. Can my home life affect my chances of having CD?

4. What are some of the symptoms of conduct disorder?

5. Am I past the point of normal risk taking?

6. How is CD diagnosed?

7. How is CD treated?

8. Where can I go to get help?

9. Do I need medication to treat conduct disorder?

10. Does my choice of friends affect my CD?

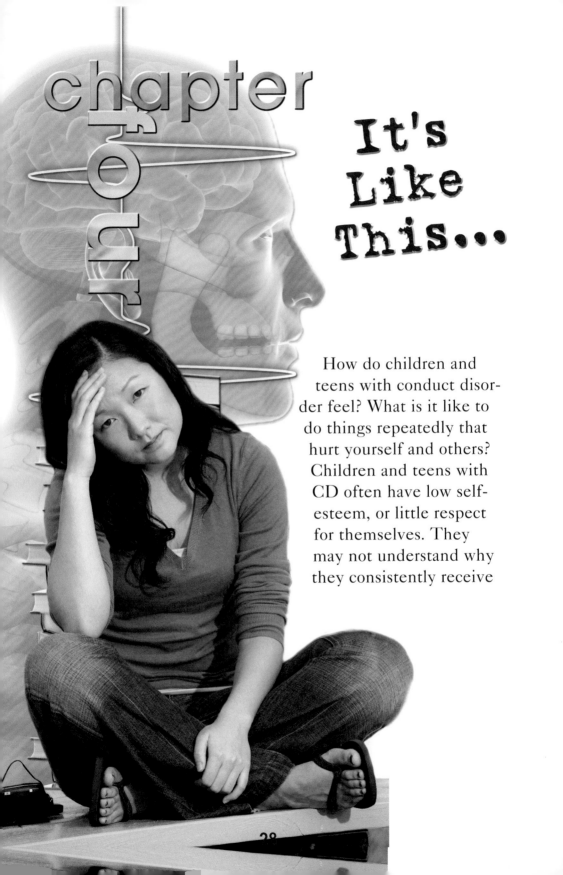

chapter four

It's Like This...

How do children and teens with conduct disorder feel? What is it like to do things repeatedly that hurt yourself and others? Children and teens with CD often have low self-esteem, or little respect for themselves. They may not understand why they consistently receive negative feedback for their behavior. As their actions toward others worsen, some teens with conduct disorder become isolated. Their family and friends no longer want to be with them because they fear for their own safety. In other cases, teens with CD may gravitate toward other people with antisocial behaviors and commit serious crimes, such as robbery or rape.

Teens who have CD usually feel intense anger, which often results in physical aggression. Imagine that you are a teen with CD. You ask your parents if you can stay out late and they say no. You become so angry at hearing "no" that you throw a chair through the window. Then you physically attack your mother. Each time you receive a "no," you react this way or worse. As a teen with conduct disorder, you exhibit a loss of control that hurts others. You may not even feel badly for your mother or your family. You do not understand how your mother feels about being hit or how your family feels at the destruction of their home. This disconnect encourages repetitive inappropriate behavior.

That you reacted by throwing the chair shows another part of conduct disorder: poor impulse control. Imagine having less control over your reactions. Rather than thinking through consequences, you react in ways that are often harmful. You may even search for ways to justify your loss of control by blaming others. "You made me do it," you tell your mother, "because you said no." You are irritable and anxious, which increases your chances of blowing up. You grew up hearing your teacher say, "Use words" to settle a conflict. But you prefer your

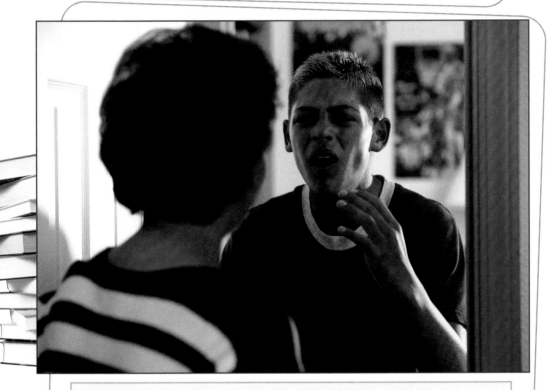

Teens who have conduct disorder can display anger, poor impulse control, and little remorse. The lack of regret hampers this individual's opportunities to learn proper behavior.

fists. You would rather hit someone to make a point. You do not show remorse for the physical and emotional pain that you cause others. This lack of guilt or regret hinders your chances of learning appropriate behavior.

There are other circumstances that affect how you feel as a teen with CD. For example, some students with conduct disorder have learning challenges. This difficulty may increase your frustration, as it takes more time and effort to learn the same material as your peers. Suppose your school sends you to the resource room for additional instruction. This action may help your learning, but it can also make you feel more isolated from your class. Another example is coming from an abusive home. Being abused can make you feel violated, embarrassed, unworthy, angry, and depressed. It can also increase the severity of your conduct disorder by modeling aggressive and violent behavior and increasing levels of frustration, anger, and irritability.

As a teen with CD, your judgment is impaired. When faced with normal risk-taking pressures, you repeatedly engage in increasing levels of risky behavior. These actions make you more likely to abuse alcohol and other drugs. Your risky behavior also pushes you toward a peer group that can influence you negatively (for instance, encouraging drug use). Remember that truancy can be an early warning sign of conduct disorder. Imagine having so many unexcused absences from school that you decide to drop out. Your chances of going to college or finding a job just decreased. This has long-term financial, social, and health costs. Today's decisions affect tomorrow's options. Teens with CD have fewer options.

Now suppose that you are teen with a serious case of conduct disorder. What began as hitting your mother, killing the neighbor's cat, and setting your friend's car on fire has escalated to raping a person whom you met at a party. She pressed charges. At first you denied doing it. Then you claim that she asked for it. You are convicted. The legal system finds that you have broken the law, violated someone else's rights, and need to go to jail as a consequence. You spend the next few years in jail. How do you feel as a teen with CD who committed this crime? How will this shape the rest of your life?

What About the Others?

Now consider that you're one of the people dealing with a teen who has conduct disorder. Maybe you are the parent who must react to and treat your child's mental disorder. You are scared by your child's actions and worried that his or her behavior will worsen. You watch in horror as he or she hurts animals. You ask your child if he or she feels remorse, and you become upset when none is shown. You can't understand how someone, especially your child, can't feel badly for someone that he or she has hurt. How is this possible? You consult friends and family members. Some respond with, "Kids will be kids." But others are equally disturbed. You cannot ignore the feeling inside of you that something is seriously wrong, and you reach out for help.

Being a parent of a child or teen with CD can be embarrassing and isolating, especially in school and social settings. Imagine being constantly called by your child's school because your child is disruptive in class. Reports include bullying other students, being excessively aggressive, and skipping school. You try to work with the professionals to address this situation, but your child increasingly acts out. Word of your child's actions spreads, and other children do not want to play or hang out with him or her. Some parents even try to give you advice, stating that

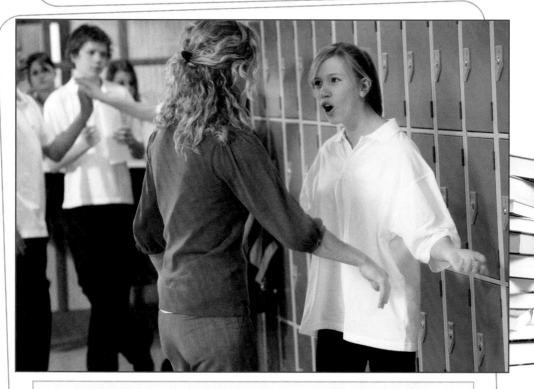

Imagine if you were a teacher who is constantly annoyed by the troubles that a student with CD causes during or between classes and worried that the student would injure another student. Teaching or parenting a teen with CD is challenging.

your child has behavioral problems because you did not raise him or her properly. They don't understand that your child's behavior is partly the result of a mental disorder.

Helplessness is another emotion that you may feel as the parent of a CD child or teen. Routine parenting or regular forms of discipline often don't work. Giving your child a "time out" only makes his or her behavior worse, as the isolation and frustration grow into more anger.

Telling your child "no" results in physical violence. You feel physically threatened by his or her presence, worried that your teen may explode and physically attack you or another family member without warning. Finally, you may search for other places to house your child—such as with family members who are willing to accept the responsibility or a therapeutic residential facility—to ensure your immediate family's safety.

Now imagine that you are another person affected by a child or teen with conduct disorder. Maybe you are a classmate who was physically attacked. Or maybe you are the neighbor whose pet was tortured to death. You may be the teacher who is persistently frustrated by disruptions and fears that the student with CD will become more physical. You may be the sister or brother of a teen with conduct disorder, and you are suffering in silence watching the violence, hearing the arguments, and becoming fearful for your safety. Some of the worst cases involve being the victim of a crime committed by a person with conduct disorder, such as murder or sexual assault.

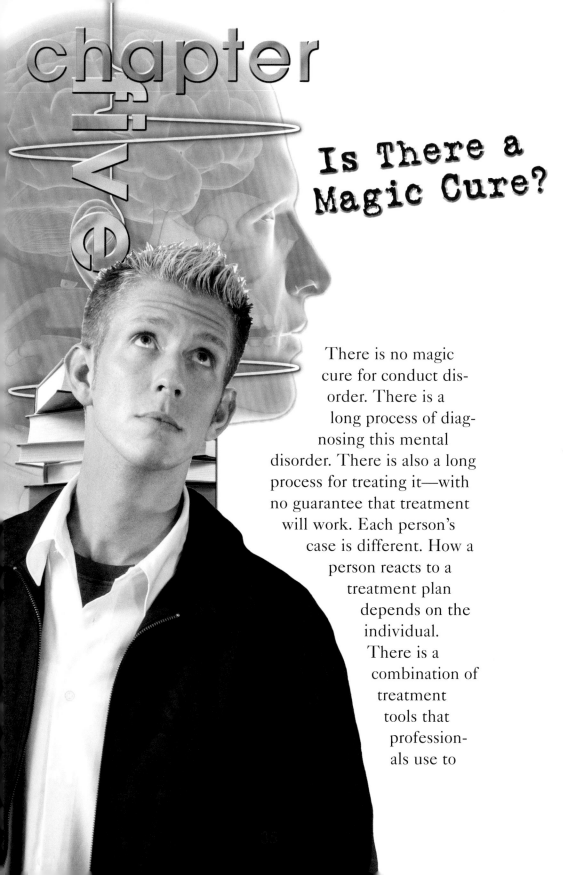

Is There a Magic Cure?

There is no magic
cure for conduct dis-
order. There is a
long process of diag-
nosing this mental
disorder. There is also a long
process for treating it—with
no guarantee that treatment
will work. Each person's
case is different. How a
person reacts to a
treatment plan
depends on the
individual.
There is a
combination of
treatment
tools that
profession-
als use to

help children and teens with CD. It is a collective effort, with caregivers, parents, and school staff working together to implement a multileveled treatment approach.

Caregivers are an important part of the treatment process. They include parent(s), grandparents, aunts, uncles, or others directly involved in the daily care of a child or teen with conduct disorder. Professionals provide parents with management training and family therapy that consists of:

- Encouraging appropriate behavior (for example, using positive reinforcement)
- Developing effective discipline tools
- Conveying clear connections between behavior and consequences
- Teaching and encouraging nondefensive, positive, effective, and direct communication
- Building trust between the conduct disorder patient and caregivers

Through the development of these skills and relationships, a child or teen can receive many benefits. He or she can link appropriate behavior with rewards and inappropriate behavior with negative consequences. For example, suppose that a child or teen receives positive reinforcement (such as earning good grades or receiving positive feedback) for attending school. Then he or she is more likely to repeat this action. If the same child or teen consistently loses privileges for skipping school, he or she may be less likely to skip school. Children and teens with conduct disorder have more difficulty making the connection between their behavior and consequences, but consistent rules over time may improve this process.

Remember that people with CD often feel isolated, sad, and upset from negative feedback. Caregivers may also feel frustrated, angry, and upset. These emotions can further break down the lines of positive communication between everyone. Psychologists and psychiatrists can open these lines by encouraging word choices and actions that perpetuate a positive environment free from defensive participants. For example, therapists might encourage people to express their feelings without placing blame on others. Positive interaction between people with CD and their caregivers also lays the foundation for trusting relationships. Children and teens with conduct disorder often lie, and it takes time for trust to build.

There are also therapy treatments specifically for patients with CD. Many children or teens receive peer or individual therapy to work through behavioral challenges and develop more appropriate behavioral patterns. Peer groups provide social skills training, where children and teens can learn appropriate social behavior, responses, and coping mechanisms. They can also develop and practice problem-solving skills that incorporate appropriate behavior.

Cognitive behavioral therapy (CBT) is one kind of therapy that helps encourage behavioral changes. CBT examines the connection between thoughts, feelings, and behavior. It seeks to improve thought processes and coping mechanisms by focusing on the thinking that leads to destructive behavior. It is an interactive therapy that comes with homework and outside practice exercises. Dialectical behavior therapy (DBT) is another

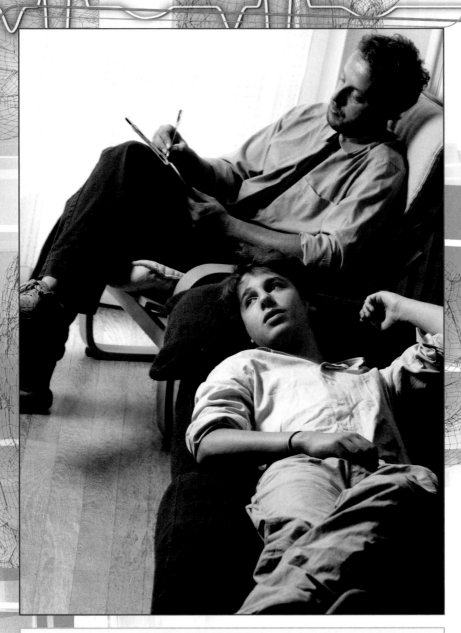

Part of the treatment process for conduct disorder
includes individual therapy sessions.

type of therapy. It looks at both biological and environmental factors that create challenges in managing emotions. DBT replaces ineffective coping mechanisms with effective ones.

For example, consider a teen with conduct disorder who often skips school. CBT would focus on what the teen is thinking that causes this action. Maybe the teen has learning issues and few friends. The teen skips school because these challenges make him or her feel worthless (have low self-esteem). A CBT therapist might replace the thought of "I am worthless" with "I have value." A DBT therapist would help the teen be mindful of his or her actions and their consequences. This professional would encourage the teen to identify contributing factors to the problem and impediments to change. Finally, the DBT therapist would encourage alternative behavior aimed at the goal of attending school.

Mental Illnesses and Medication

Many children and teens exhibit symptoms of more than one mental, emotional, or behavioral disorder. Consider a teen with CD who is also very anxious and hyperactive. This behavior may encourage a doctor to also consider diagnoses of generalized anxiety disorder (GAD) and attention deficit disorder (ADD) or attention-deficit/hyperactivity disorder (ADHD). In treating a patient with medication, doctors treat the symptoms. There are no particular medications for conduct disorder, but doctors may prescribe medications typically used for other disorders.

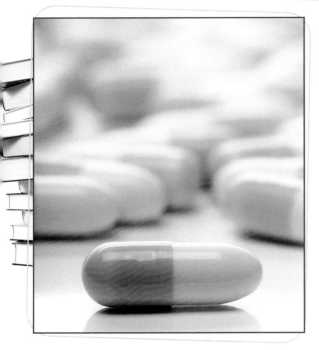

Medications are often used to decrease symptoms of conduct disorder.

Common ADHD medications, such as Ritalin and Dexedrine, have been effective in treating CD patients. These medications can decrease aggression in children and teens and make them calmer. Many people with conduct disorder are also depressed. Causes may be biological (chemical makeup of the body) or environmental (such as reactions to isolation and negative feedback). Antidepressants, such as Wellbutin and Prozac, can relieve this depression. These medications can also reduce impulsivity and aggression.

There are other medications used to reduce aggressive outbursts and impulsive behavior, such as lithium, clonidine, Dilantin, Depakene, and Tegretol. Symptom reduction allows patients to be more receptive to therapy and to apply new behavioral patterns and coping mechanisms. It can also result in better functioning at home, school, and social settings because there are fewer physical outbursts and other destructive behaviors. All of these medications are prescribed and monitored by doctors. Caregivers must report side effects, which can include drowsiness, vomiting, seizures, and restlessness.

Getting Help

Suppose the mother of a teen with CD takes her son to a psychiatrist. She provides his developmental and behavioral histories. She describes both home and school settings and asks teachers, administrators, and the school psychologist to provide reports. The mom mentions that her son is highly intelligent, with emotional and behavioral challenges. She has recently enrolled him in a social skills group. This teen is young, and his mother wants to treat his CD. She has another child at home and local family support.

The psychiatrist helps this mother develop a treatment plan that includes medication and therapy. She administers the medication and takes her son for needed follow-up blood work. She reports side effects and behavioral changes associated with the medication. Her son no longer feels intense anger. His mother finds a DBT therapist, who helps him become aware of his actions and their consequences. Together, the people in this teen's life develop a treatment plan that is consistently applied throughout his home and school environments. Over time, he begins to develop more appropriate behavioral patterns.

How common is this teen's reaction to his treatment plan? Unfortunately, CD remains a serious disorder that is difficult to treat. It affects millions of children and teens.

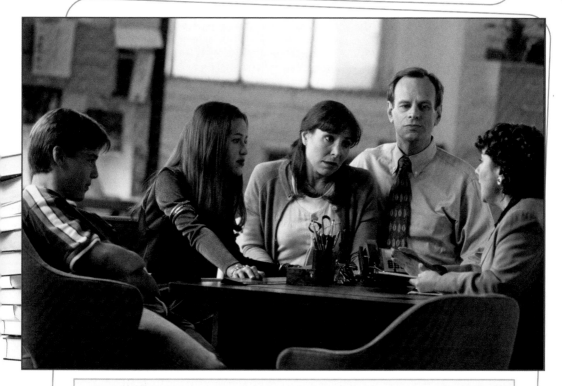

Treating a teen with conduct disorder requires many people working together.

Chances for recovery are higher when treated at an earlier age and with a multileveled approach (medical, mental, and educational) by caregivers, doctors, and school staff. Appropriate treatment of coexisting disorders, along with early diagnosis and treatment and continual help and encouragement, may improve the future of an individual who has conduct disorder.

abuse To hurt or injure physically or emotionally.

aggression Violent behavior toward others.

cognitive behavioral therapy (CBT) A therapeutic approach that examines the connection between thoughts, feelings, and behavior.

conduct disorder (CD) A mental disorder that involves aggression toward people or animals, destruction of property, lying or theft, and/or the serious violation of rules.

depression A mental state involving extreme sadness and feelings of inadequacy.

dialectal behavior therapy (DBT) A therapeutic approach that looks at both biological and environmental factors contributing to challenges with managing emotions.

empathy An ability to relate to someone else's feelings.

impulsivity The tendency to act on desire instead of thought.

mental disorder An emotional and behavioral challenge that requires psychiatric care.

oppositional defiant disorder (ODD) A milder form of conduct disorder.

psychiatrist A doctor who specializes in mental illnesses.

psychologist A person trained in dealing with the mind and emotions.

remorse Regret for a wrong action.

self-esteem Respect for yourself.

suicide Killing oneself on purpose.

truancy An unexcused absence from school.

violation A lack of respect for someone's rights, privacy, or feelings.

American Academy of Child & Adolescent Psychiatry
(AACAP)
3615 Wisconsin Avenue NW
Washington, DC 20016-3007
(202) 966-7300
Web site: http://www.aacap.org
This leading American professional medical association
helps patients with mental illnesses and their families.

Canadian Academy of Child and Adolescent Psychiatry
(CACAP)
701-141 Laurier Avenue West
Ottawa, ON K1P 5J3
Canada
(613) 288-0408
Web site: http://www.cacap-acpea.org
This national organization is dedicated to furthering the
mental health of children, youth, and families.

Canadian Mental Health Association, Ontario (CMHA)
180 Dundas Street West, Suite 2301
Toronto, ON M5G 1Z8
Canada
(416) 977-5580
(800) 875-6213
Web site: http://www.ontario.cmha.ca
This nonprofit organization aims to make mental health
possible for everyone.

Mental Health America (MHA)
2000 North Beauregard Street, 6th Floor

Alexandria, VA 22311
(800) 969-6642
Web site: http://www.nmha.org
The MHA encourages health care access for people with
mental and substance abuse conditions.

National Alliance on Mental Illness (NAMI)
3803 North Fairfax Drive, Suite 100
Arlington, VA 22203
(800) 950-NAMI (6264)
Web site: http://www.nami.org
The NAMI advocates for mental health services, treatments, and research.

National Institute of Mental Health (NIMH)
6001 Executive Boulevard, Room 8184, MSC 9663
Bethesda, MD 20892-9663
(301) 443-4513
Web site: http://www.nimh.nih.gov
The NIMH furthers the understanding and treatment of
mental illness through basic and clinical research.

Web Sites

Due to the changing nature of Internet links, Rosen
Publishing has developed an online list of Web sites
related to the subject of this book. This site is updated
regularly. Please use this link to access the list:

http://www.rosenlinks.com/TMH/Cond

Bancroft, Lundy. *When Dad Hurts Mom: Helping Your Children Heal the Wounds of Witnessing Abuse.* New York, NY: Berkley Books, 2004.

Bancroft, Lundy. *Why Does He Do That? Inside the Minds of Angry and Controlling Men.* New York, NY: Berkley Books, 2002.

Bellenir, Karen. *Mental Health Information for Teens: Health Tips About Mental Wellness and Mental Illness.* 3rd ed. Farmington Hills, MI: Gale Cengage Learning, 2010.

Biegel, Gina. *The Stress Reduction Workbook for Teens: Mindfulness Skills to Help You Deal with Stress.* Oakland, CA: Instant Help, 2010.

Carlson, Richard, Jr. *Please Stop Smiling.* Seattle, WA: CreateSpace, 2012.

Gilgun, Jane. F. *Lemons or Lemonade: An Anger Workbook for Kids.* Seattle, WA: CreateSpace, 2012.

Hart, K. J., A. J. Finch, Jr., and W. M. Nelson III. *Conduct Disorder: A Practitioner's Guide to Comparative Treatments.* New York, NY: Springer Publishing, 2006.

Martinez, Katherine A., and Michael A. Tompkins. *My Anxious Mind: A Teen's Guide to Managing Anxiety and Panic.* Washington, DC: Magination Press, 2009.

Mash, Eric J., and David A. Wolfe. *Abnormal Child Psychology.* Independence, KY: Cengage Learning, 2012.

Matthys, Walter, and John E. Lochman. *Oppositional Defiant Disorder and Conduct Disorder in Children.* Hoboken, NJ: Wiley, 2009.

Van Dijk, Sheri. *Don't Let Your Emotions Run Your Life for Teens: Dialectical Behavior Therapy Skills for Helping You Manage Mood Swings, Control Angry Outbursts, and Get Along with Others.* Oakland, CA: Instant Help, 2011.

About the Author

Barbara Gottfried Hollander has worked in many areas of education as a curriculum developer, course writer, classroom teacher, and private learning consultant in both mainstream and special-needs schools. She has written numerous books for teens, including *Addiction*, part of the Understanding Brain Diseases and Disorders series.

Photo Credits

Designer: Nicole Russo; Editor: Kathy Kuhtz Campbell; Photo Researcher: Marty Levick